Panic Attacks: Cause and Treatment

How to get rid of it in 3 days!!!

John Bradford

John Bradford

Table of Content

Introduction

I want to thank you and congratulate you for downloading the book, *"How To Stop Panic Attacks In 3 Minutes Or Less: A Practical, No-Nonsense Guide To Make It 'A History'."*

In this book, I want to be your guardian angel. To tap your shoulder and show you the exact steps you need to take so that you can end panic attacks.

Ending panic attack is easy if you know what to do. I am qualified to tell you this because I experienced my first panic attacks when I was the age of 18 years.

It was a dreadful experience that I cannot wish for anyone, especially teenagers.

An adult can control it, but when you are a teenager at the age of 14 or 16, it can be a hard experience.

Because the fear and thoughts of dying won't get away from your mind that easy. Even if somebody handed you advice, it looks too hard to be true.

You feel that the person telling you doesn't understand what you are going through. This book has some good practical suggestion that anybody can take. I wanted to publish a book that cuts across all people. That means, if you are 30 or 14 years and panic attacks Is still a problem, you will benefit a lot from my experiences towards the healing process.

In this book, you will learn the following.

  x   Understand The Science Of Panic Attacks(How They Happen)

x 7 Dumbest Mistakes People Do When They Have Panic Attack

x 2 Things You Need To Do Immediately When Panic Attacks Strikes

x Medication And Treatment That Can Help You Cope Up With It.

x 5 Healthy Lifestyle Habits You Can Start Today To Make Panic Attacks A Thing Of The Past

All this information are as a result of my experience of what I have gone through to solve this problem.

When I started applying the two techniques in chapter three, I was able to calm this condition in 3 minutes. The first day it looked „kinda" hard, but the more I got used to it, the more I was able to calm the situation.

I came to believe that if I controlled my breath properly, I could bring this process to stop. Fortunately, when you look at chapter 3, I go into details of breathing pattern you need to follow.

Plus the exact steps you need to do. I guarantee you that if you follow this steps panic attacks will be a thing of the past.

In chapter two, I also go into more details of the mistakes that you need to avoid. What I have come to realize is that these mistakes hold most people back towards the recovery process.

In fact, most people associate these same mistakes with recovery which is the exact opposite. You are just making the condition worse day by day.

In the last chapter, I show you the healthy lifestyle habits that you need to incorporate in your life.

If you follow this healthy lifestyle habit, for 3 months, your life would have changed for good.

You may be asking...Why I have included this lifestyle habits in this book.

Simple:

A Panic attack is not a disease, and it has never been a disease. Panic attacks are lifestyle conditions. And like any other lifestyle conditions, it can be cured or healed by adopting certain habits in your life.

These habits are meant to bring you back to reality towards the healing process, especially the first tip that I provide you. It is helpful, and it will make you recover fast.

It is the same tip that I am sharing with you today. I am sure if you keep a regular schedule even if you don't follow my other suggestion, you could get the results that you want within some few months.

Enough of the introduction... Now let us turn to our first chapter, to get a clue of what actually panic attacks...And the psychological process that happens the moment panic attacks takes place.

When you know that...You will know to calm and relax your body.

John Bradford

Understand the Science of Panic Attacks (How They Happen)

"Oh no! It is going on again! Not again! I think I need to get out of here! The day before it happen here, I can't have it here; I will embarrass myself in front of these people. Quick, quick, quick!"

Do you occasionally see yourself in this situation?

These are signs that you have a panic attack.

Sadly, 6 million of adults in America today, suffer from panic anxiety and disorder that is 2.7% of the population.

My goal today is to make sure that this number decreases, that is to mean, at the end of this short ebook you will be able to get rid of panic attacks for the rest of your life.

A panic attack doesn't have to distract your daily life. Okay, maybe you may be asking...

What is a panic attack?

In short...It is a particular surge of intense fear that overwhelms the body and mind such that it makes the person think they are going to die or have a heart attack.

For you to understand panic attacks, you need to know how your body reacts, when you experience this conditions.

That is to say, the science of panic attacks. Here is a simple explanation.

When panic attacks strike, Adrenaline causes the heart to pump more blood to the major muscles of your body so that you can run fast.

At the same time, you also get extra strength in your arm. This additional blood goes to your brain to give you that extra urge to respond to emergencies.

It only takes 3 minutes for your brain and your body to be fully adrenalized with more blood to your legs and arms.

In that short time, you experience your heart pumping and more blood flowing throughout the body.

The more your adrenal glands keep receiving more emergency message, the more it produces more adrenaline.

Once your brain stops getting this message, your adrenal glands stop producing more adrenal glands.

3 minutes is the only time your adrenal glands needs to fill your body with adrenal responses.

At the same time, it also takes 3 minutes for your body to stop the adrenaline reaction.

For people who have developed a panic disorder, this condition can take 10 minutes or more if it is not controlled.

The bottom line.

It is not a life and death situation as most people put. It is a condition that can be managed with proper care.

The fact is.

You won't die

So, how do you know if you have panic attacks or what are the exact signs and symptoms of panic attacks?

Well, here are the signs and symptoms of it:

x   Fear of going crazy

x   Fear of death

x   Feeling like you will have a stroke that may make you disable

x   Chest pains

x   A racing heart

x   Feeling like you have difficult to breath

x   Tingling or shaking of the arms, legs or hands

x   Dizziness and lightheadedness.

These are the common signs and symptoms that you people who have panic attacks experience. But what makes a person have this panic attack?

There is no scientific explanation for what makes people have panic attacks.

But here is what we know... When people start experiencing fear of something. Let say they start thinking of something going to happen to their loved ones.

Or they start thinking that they forgot to lock the door when they are out, and they start thinking maybe a burglar will break into their house.

In short...they develop a fear of something that is not going to happen and they get worried. When such situation clouds their mind that is when the adrenal glands start producing this adrenaline to give the person more strength so that they can run fast.

These are not only situations that trigger panic attacks in people. In a study done by the American Journal Of Medicine, individuals who take coffee, smoke or drink are also likely to get panic attacks.

Even watching horror movies, reality TV shows and drama can trigger panic attacks.

In simple terms, something that can scare you, or make you sad has a potential effect of making you sad.

Now, what are the long-term effect of panic attacks? If you stay with this condition for a long time, you may develop panic disorder.

You may not be able to do your daily chores in life. Or you may succumb to agoraphobia.

In the next chapter, you are about to learn the common mistake that people make when they have these conditions.

7 Mistakes You Should Avoid When You Have Panic Attacks

"You are today where your thoughts have brought you; you will be tomorrow where your thoughts take you." ~James Allen

Could it be true that the reason why you have panic attacks is that you are making certain mistakes that make the condition worse each and every single day?

I was a happy a child until everything came to a stand still when I had my first panic attacks.

It was a horrifying experience. Worst of all it is that it happened during the night.

I felt intense fear, even explaining things to my girlfriend were difficult. But what I knew at the back of my mind was that the experience I had resembles animal-like horror.

From that day onwards I had a series of those attacks. It robbed me of my life; my girlfriend broke up with me because I couldn't control the situation.

The only people who were there for me were my parents and therapist.

I lost all friends, and I was lonely most of my time. But later in life at the age of 24 years, things started to change.

That is when I began to realize that the things I was doing to control the situation were completely wrong.

I was doing the same things over and over again, with no real results.

As it turns out, this is the exact things people who have panic attacks are constantly doing to get rid of these conditions.

So here are the dumbest mistakes that you should avoid doing. I guarantee you that when you eliminate these mistakes, you will get excellent results in your recovery.

Mistake #1: Resisting

It is logical.

It is human nature.

The moment you start feeling sad about something or experience depression, the easiest thing that you do is to try to change your mood so that you are feeling good.

But, trying to convince your mind out of it, would not work. The more you try to resist it, the more you think about the bad feelings.

The results.

Your brain starts to detect this as emergencies, and the adrenal gland starts producing more adrenaline. After a short period you start sweating, your hands start shaking, and dizziness clouds in.

Before you know it, you have another panic attack.

The truth.

You can't control it. The more you try to control it the more you will have stress, and if you are not careful, you may have another panic attack.

My therapist told me that the best way to deal with this situation is to calm and relax. Unfortunately, this is not always easy as it looks.

It is hard to be calm and relax when you have panic attacks. But my advice for you is that you need to at least try it out whenever it happens.

Fortunately, in the last section of the ebook, you will get helpful suggestions to calm and relaxation techniques to control panic attacks.

Mistake #2: Negative Thoughts And Bad Feeling.

'I can't believe this is happening again. I just need to be out of here! This is crazy. I am gonna die! I am having a stroke!

Well, when panic strikes, the only words that come out of people's mouth are negative thoughts and feeling.

You just feel that you are alone in the world. You are about to die. The negative feeling and thoughts are what keeps this condition happening to you most of the time.

It is like you are addicted to something.

The truth.

The negative feelings and thoughts are the habit pattern of the mind. In short, it is something that you can control.

But again, I will be lying to you when I say to you that it is easy. Even the most confident person in the world experience negative thoughts and feeling about things.

The only difference...Is how you manage it. You can't get rid of negative feelings, but you can control them. You can listen to them.

In this book, preferable in the next chapter, there is one powerful suggestion on how you can control negative thoughts.

Believe me, after doing these countless number of time; you will be able to control any thoughts that you may have.,

Sometimes, the mind wants you to believe what you want to believe. If you feel that you are going to die, then it will find every suggestion to convince you that it is true.

9

The mind goes to collect answers from previous experience where you have situations that resemble death.

That is why people who get panic attacks in a supermarket always think that they should not go to that supermarket. The reason...They will get panic attacks.

Or if they got a panic attack in a crowded place, they will surely avoid crowded places.

But what you are doing here is not solving the problem, you are making these thoughts become a reality in your mind.

If you train your mind to have positive feelings and thoughts, then panic attacks are going to be a history.

Mistake #3: Comparing Your Past Life With the Present

I believe you remember how normal your life was before you start getting panic attacks.

Right now, am sure that you feel awkward.

What I have released in my recovery journey from panic attacks is that comparing your past life with the present is not the solution.

If you want to get a chance to recover, you have to forget the past. Just say the past is the past. I can't change things.

You see, the moment you start comparing the past with the present, you are worsening the situation.

You are not accepting the situation. Acceptance is the healing process towards a panic attack.

If you start to accept it, you start living in the present and making a positive change in your life.

Any therapist will tell you how acceptance is the good remedy when it comes to curing panic attacks.

Mistake #4: Question! Question! Question!

Why! Why! Why me?

Why am I the only person having this? Has the Lord forsaken me? Why can't I have a normal life just like other people?

Six years back, this pointless question kept clouding my mind whenever I was alone.

The truth of the matter.

They didn't help. They made me sad. They made me lose that special person in my life.

Questions like this will make you remain with panic attacks for the rest of your life. Even if you said them, there is no clear answer.

The only answer you get is sadness, depression, and anxiety. Instead, you should ask what I am going to do about it. At least this way, your mind will find a clue to how you can solve the situations.

Mistake #5: Believing Your Fears; That Things Will Happen

The thoughts of dying.

The thought of heart attack.

The thoughts of stroke.

If you believe that you have these things, although you have no heart conditions, you are storming the situation.

As I said earlier, the mind wants you to believe these things are real. That they are going to happen to you.

By that, you don't even need to make a mistake that of saying that you are not going to die. Or, I will not end up in a heart attack.

Saying such phrases is like you are sprouting negative thoughts, and these thoughts will make you believe such fears.

Some people will tell you just to ignore it...You can't ignore what is inside you. You can only substitute these feelings and emotions to something else...And the fears will go.

Let me give you a little example.

It is so easy to tell a person who is an addict to smoking that they need to quit smoking.

You take them to rehab, and it doesn't work. What I have discovered is that you can't change bad habits, but you can substitute a habit.

For example, a smoke addict can try substituting smoking to jogging. When you feel like smoking, you start to jog.

13

You see, doing things like this makes you forget tobacco use. As for panic attacks, I have found a good useful you way of distracting your mind whenever it happens.

You will find it in the next chapter. So continue reading on.

Mistake #6: Seeking Solution From Outside.

I am not against this.

If I am against this, I will be saying that it doesn't make sense to consult a therapist.

But what do I mean by this... The solution to this problem lies with you. You have the capability. You don't need an outside source to solve this issue.

Here is what I discovered.

To end this, you don't have to believe that your therapist is the solution or certain medication is the remedy.

You just need to have the drive and motivation to finish this. You need to face it from inside.

Only then will you have the chance to make this history.

That explains why some people end up having panic attacks for the rest of their life. It is because of lack motivation or drive.

Their motivation depends on another person telling them what to do.

One thing is you need to realize about motivation is that...If it comes from an outside source, it usually fades away. But when it comes inside you with a couple of determination and will power is strong.

If you can get that courage and motivation that you want to end this. That it has to stop. And you are going to do anything that is possible under the sun to stop it.

John Bradford

Then my friend you will have no fear. The enemy lies within and is making you believe that you can fight it from outside. Kill the enemy from within and you will end this.

Mistake #7: Wanting To Be Alone

You've heard it.

'An idle mind is the devil's workshop.'

Or, 'Idle hands are the devil's tools.'

When I had panic attacks, I thought that if I am alone, maybe, I will be happy. Or I will not get it.

But the opposite happened.

Negative feelings and thoughts started clouding my mind. A sense of unworthiness, self-pity, and low self-esteem is all I ever achieved.

Later on, I realized... That being alone doesn't help any inch in my recovery.

So here is what I started doing.

I started spending time with positive people; I started spending time in social gatherings where people were having fun.

But if there is one thing that you need to come out from is spending your time with negative people.

Now, you be asking...Where I do spend my time with positive people. Do worry; I have included a list of places you can find positive people in this book.

Your job is to continue read... In the last section, you will find all that.

If you can get rid of these 7 dumbest mistakes, you will be on your quick way to recover fast.

I believe in the next 40 days or some few months you will start getting positive results that you can be proud. You don't have to stay with these conditions for the rest of your life.

Okay...Now that you know the mistakes that you need to avoid. It is a time you learn what to do when panic attacks strike. I believe this is the most dreadful situations.

In the next section of the books, you are about to learn...

2 Things You Need To Do Immediately When You Panic Attacks Strikes

You feel it.

You sense it.

You see it coming.

You start thinking...Should I run or should get away from it. What if! What if! What if!

If you give in as I have said earlier, you are not helping. Panic attacks is a habit pattern of the mind. How you respond to it when it happens is what will save you.

Fortunately... I want to show you what I did every time that I had panic attacks.

It was a big life saver to me. I believe by the end of this section...You will know what exactly you need to do.

First.

Something of the things I did may sound scary. Or you feel that these things are won't help the situation.

But here is the truth of the matter.

Some of my suggestions I got them from reading self-help books and they helped me.

After reading a countless number of books that is when it dawn on me that panic attack is a condition. That, when you control the 19 input that you give your mind...You can get rid of a panic attack for good.

My point.

The battle begins in the mind. There is where everything lies. Train your mind to face it with courage and make it look for the solution.

So here is what you need to do...

Mind Solution #1: Get A Journal Or Panic Book

Your mind can be a big bank for storing all the negative emotions and thoughts you have.

The more you live each day with unpleasant thought the more your brain stores them. The more your mind connects with the problem. The more your mind forces you to believe that everything that is happening to you is real.

The good news.

You can train your mind to connect with your emotions and find solutions to problem like panic attacks.

Here is the first thing to do.

You need to empty these thoughts so that your brain finds the solution to them. And there is no better way of doing this rather than documenting your feelings in the journal.

When you have panic attacks, write down what you feel. If it is negative, write it down.

If you are feelings that you are going to die...Write I am just about to die in the next few minutes.

Don't leave the pen hanging in the middle of your writing. Continue adding more sentences, never mind about the spelling or the grammar.

You will come to realize that after sometimes you start feeling calm and more relaxed. You will start gaining clarity with your feelings and thoughts.

You will begin to get an understanding of yourself.

The good news...

The more you understand yourself, the more your mind starts getting solutions.

When I started journaling every feeling I had during panic attacks... My mind started giving me more solution to the problem.

At one time I got the idea that... To end panic attacks I need to read books on the subject at least a day. I began to read panic books, self-help books, happiness books and abundance books.

What I discovered later is that by journaling my thoughts, I was like sending my mind to find the solution.

Now, journaling may look like easy on paper. But it is not. In fact, you may feel awkward about it, because it is not your thing.

But if you want to get good results and adopt it in your life you need 40 days...And by the end of it, you will get used to it.

Let me distract you away from the subject a little.

If you look at any person, who has been successful they will tell you how writing your goal each single day can be crucial.

The truth is.

Writing your goals each single day keeps you closer to reach your goals... And since your mind is creative it will keep finding new solutions every time to keep you ahead.

Same applies to panic attacks, just start writing your feelings and thoughts down and you will start seeing the miracle.

Mind Solution #2: The Kind Of Breathing You Need To Do.

You see, panic attacks is a result of over breathing or what is typically known as hyperventilation.

That is why you see people who have panic attacks feel that they are running out of breath. Which is the opposite of what happens?

Feeling like you are running out of breath is as a result of you having excess oxygen in your body.

Now, to use this excess oxygen, your body needs a certain amount of carbon dioxide in the body.

Fortunately, you can learn to control your breath. There two ways you can counter hyperventilation.

First method.

Take a slow breath of 10 to 15 seconds. Do this repeatedly and you calm the hyperventilation situation. In the process, you will be able to get the amount of oxygen your body needs to calm the situation.

Or.

The other way can be for you, take a brisk walk or jog while you are breathing through your nose, which calms the process of hyperventilation.

Note:

You need to get the first method correctly. When doing this, you should take a slow breath, not deep breath.

A deep breath can worsen the condition. Just take a slow breath of 10 to 15 seconds

Second method.

Here you need to learn about how to do a particular type of breathing called belly or diaphragm breathing. It helps a lot.

What you need to know before you begin:

To get good results with this method, you need to take a longer time exhaling the air. Like 10 seconds exhaling and 5 seconds inhaling. This will balance the oxygen and carbon dioxide ratio in the body and eventually you will calm down

There is a biological law that states that if you breathe in this way, your body will have to come to a point and relax. It will have no choices left.

Here the exact steps you need to take:

Step One.

Take one hand and place it in your belt line. Take the other and place it on your chest. This will help you know which area you are using to breathe.

Step Two:

Close your eyes and this time, I need you to focus on your breath. Fortunately, closing your eyes will make your mind focus on what you are doing instead of what you are feeling.

Step Three:

Take a count of 6 when you are breathing in and take a count of 12 when you are breathing out. It is that simple. When you carry out this process, I repeat, take a slow breath, not deep.

Step Four:

When you are breathing out, take a count of 12, make sure that your shoulders and the muscles of your upper body, relax very slowly. Don't give a sigh, what you need is to make it look like you are relaxing your muscles.

Step Five:

Repeat the same situation until you are fully relaxed from the situation

One more thing.

It is not easy to do this type of breathing at first, but you need to give it a try if you want to get good results from your condition.

If you learn how to do these two methods, you can get rid of panic attacks in three minutes or less.

Although the first time you will experience some difficulty, rest assured that the more effort you put, the higher your chances of ending panic attacks.

Now, you may be wondering, apart from these two methods... What about medication. That is what you will learn in the next section... Turn the page on...

Medication And Treatment That Can Help

This section of the book will be short because I believe most of the information and guideline can be found when you consult a therapist.

A therapist can tell you the kind of drugs that you need to take. As for me, during the early stages of panic attacks I was advised to take antidepressants and Benzodiazepines.

Am sure if you go through the internet, you will find lots of information on the drugs that you need to take.

But first.

You need a thorough medical examination and evaluation. Consider this option of seeking a therapist, if you see that you cannot manage the situation on your own.

Or if you still have some fears in you.

One more thing:

Drugs are a temporary solution to getting rid of a panic attack. Drugs also have side effects that is why I would prefer you not to become a dependent on them.

You can also start taking supplements they can help to ease up the situation. Personally, I like to take Tiens Supplement from China.

If you study Traditional Chinese Medicine (TCM), you will know how good their supplements are.

About the supplements, this is just an opinion because of the good results that I have seen happened to me.

I know they are, some people opposed to taking supplements from China, but if you study their history well, you will get to know how they are effective. At first, I was skeptical about the idea, but I had to do research and find things by myself.

What I realized is that they have made a tremendous improvement in the field of medicine than American and Europe.

5 Healthy Lifestyle Habit You Can Start Today To Make Panic Attacks A Thing Of The Past

Here is the good news that is going to change the way you view panic attacks.

It is a lifestyle condition like heart attacks and diabetes.

That means... You can end it.

For me, when I started this regular activity, I was startled on the results I was having. Instead of having three regular panic attacks in a week, I started having them one in a week.

And it went to one after every two weeks, then one in a month. It until my big break came when I was able to go through the year without panic attacks.

Up to this day, I still do some of the activities that I am about to list here. But for health reasons.

Lifestyle Tip #1: Take A Yoga Class(Here is Why)

I remember telling you earlier lots about the adrenal glands and its function.

The good news is that...Yoga exercise regulates the adrenal gland. And this gland is the one that is responsible for filling your body with adrenaline, making your heart race and your whole body sweating.

Yoga also helps you to focus on the present. People who do Yoga are always able to concentrate and solve problems in life. They are always positive people.

Earlier on, I told you that you should interact with positive people. And having two or three people as friends from your Yoga class will be a great help.

In my experience, Yoga will teach how to breathe properly. It is one of the best relaxation or meditation techniques that you can do.

Lifestyle Tip #2: Regular Exercises

I really can't emphasize on how important this is...Not only to your health, but in the treatment of your panic attacks.

When I first started regular exercise, I began with swimming twice a week. Then I went to three times a week, by the end of the month I was doing daily workouts in the morning.

While in the evening, I went to my Yoga classes. But you don't have to start these two kinds of activities together. You can take one activity at a time like I did.

I started with taking Yoga in the evening, then when I got used to it for like a month. I started swimming every morning, by the end of the month I was able to combine these two activities.

Again, you don't have to take these two activities together. Just including one in your life will help you.

Lifestyle Tip #3: Have A Good Night Sleep.

Regular sleep is good for your health. If every morning you wake up with bad moods that means you rarely have a good night's sleep.

Researchers and psychologist link lack of sleep with diet. If you take a proper diet, you will have a better sleep at night.

For you take have a good sleep, you will need to take your supper 3 hours before you go to sleep. And your food has to be light. In the next tip, you will learn more about this.

Lifestyle Tip #4: Stick On A Good Diet.

You are what you eat. Your health is your greatest asset.

Those words were said by Socrates, and they apply to our life today. Eat a well-balanced diet.

Give your focus to organic food because they are rich in nutrients that will help your body.

In the evening, take light meals and take them three hours before you go to sleep. A good breakfast and a heavy lunch should be your priority.

Lifestyle Tip #5: Take Regular Hot bathtub.

Soaking your body in a hot tub for some few minutes will relieve you from the daily stress of life.

The therapeutic benefit of a hot tub can relieve you from depression and make you have a good night's sleep.

If you take 20 minutes a day soaking your body in a bathtub, you will have a peace of mind. The soothing sensation of the hot water will provide your body with wonderful massage experience.

Although there are no clinical studies that support how hot bathtub can help relieve you from panic attacks. But other studies that are there reveal that soaking your body in a bathtub can relieve you from stress, anxiety, depression and other lifestyle diseases.

According to me, I believe that soaking your body in a hot bathtub can be of help.

John Bradford

Final Thoughts

I won't say that it is easy, but what I know is that if you have the motivation and the drive you can end this.

You can make it a 'thing' of the past. You don't have to slog with this condition till you get old.

Fortunately, you are a lucky person because you have finished reading a book from somebody who has gone through the same experience and he understands what it feels like to have a panic attack.

If you become serious with Yoga, you will learn a lot about meditation and how to breath.

I urge you to try your best to end this. Not by drugs, because that is just a temporary solution. But you can take good supplements which act nutrient in your body.

I have strong belief that if you apply the suggestion in this book, even if it is only one. You will begin to see changes happening in your life.

You don't have to do all the things that I said here, but you do have to start at least with one thing, then month by month as you gain the confidence you could do other things.

That is how I started. I know how the information in this book can be overwhelming; that is why I recommend you to take one thing at a time.

If you feel like you need help that much or you have developed a disorder as a result of a series of panic attacks, you can always seek the counsel of a trained therapist.

Even if you get the therapist, as long as you are willing to do your part, you will be making big progress.

The reason why I believe that panic attacks can end... is that panic attacks are habits of mind that you form. You create a mental picture of something that is unreal. And as I have outlined earlier, if you can train your mind well.

These panic attacks can be a history. You just have to do it, and your life will change.

Thank you very much for reading this book. I believe these ideas will be of great help to you.

Conclusion

Thank you again for downloading this book!

I hope this book was able to help you to cope up with panic attack

The next step is to for you is take action.

Finally, if you enjoyed this book, then I"d like to ask you for a favor, would you be kind enough to leave a review for this book on Amazon? It"d be greatly appreciated!

Thank you and good luck!

www.ingramcontent.com/pod-product-compliance
Lightning Source LLC
Chambersburg PA
CBHW070237290526
45789CB00004B/1658